A Swing and a Miss

The Funny, Tragic, and Scary True Stories of Real Swingers

By

Audra Morgan

A Swing and a Miss: The Funny, Tragic, and Scary True Stories of Real Swingers

ISBN# **978-1495438677**

Copyright © 2014 by Audra Morgan

Audra can be contacted by email at

AudraMorganBooks@gmail.com

Table of Contents

Introduction

Last year, I put together a little memoir of my own experiences during the past five years in the swinging community. I've had more than a few people ask me, "Was that all *really* true?" I am sad to say, yes, it's all true. Not only is it all true, but there were some stories *so* tragic that I didn't include them, because my intent was to amuse and entertain, not to downright depress my readers. As I pointed out, I've also had some wonderful experiences, but the focus of the book was on the misadventures, the misfires, the absolutely confounding experiences in which one can find themselves in the wacky world of swinging.

Over the past year, I've also had the good fortune of having readers, as well as others I've been able to personally interview, share their own interesting and sometimes tragically funny anecdotes with me. It was a relief to know that these borderline insane encounters were not simply a tragedy meant to befall only me; they're apparently endemic to the community. It's a wonderful world of sexual exploration, but it's also a world which attracts all manners of weirdness, drama, and mental instability.

Please understand, these stories are not meant to discourage anyone from delving into open relationships of any kind. I'm still going strong, despite the many hiccups (to put it mildly) I've encountered. I find sexual openness to be a wonderful gift, and my husband and I will never go back to being monogamous. These stories simply give you a peek into the side of swinging that television documentaries don't show you, that erotica won't detail for you, and that most people don't casually tell their friends while discussing their weekends. So be entertained by them, and by the fact that real life is indeed often much,

much stranger than fiction. And should you decide to give swinging a try, perhaps these tales will assist you in detecting warning signs that things are not quite what you thought they were. So read it for humor, or use it as a self-help guide. Either way, I hope you enjoy. And to those of you whose stories grace the following pages, my sincerest thanks for being so open about some experiences that most people would dare not share with their best friend, much less with a stranger.

Chapter One

Sex, Lies, and Picture Collectors

One of the most common complaints from swingers is that people online, to put it quite bluntly, lie. They lie a lot. The usual suspects for such duplicity fill the thousands of pages of ads on Craigslist for "casual encounters." Many of them are picture collectors, hoping to lure people into sharing their own private x-rated photos in the hopes of meeting a compatible couple or single person. Sadly, the person at the other end simply wants to add a few naughty photos to his collection; he has no actual interest in meeting, and he is most likely not who he represents himself to be. Single men often masquerade as hot young single women looking for threesomes, or as couples looking to make a connection with other couples. Many naïve, and unfortunately, seasoned, swingers fall prey to this tactic, and who knows where all those photos end up.

Just last week, I was duped by a picture collector, and the funniest part of it all is that I was working on this chapter when it happened. Proof positive that sometimes you're not nearly as clever as you think you are. I was browsing the swingers website to which we belong, and I noticed a single woman's profile which I had not seen before. She was a paid member of the site and had two certifications from couples which verified that she was legit. So far, so good. She had a few photos up, all of which seemed perfectly normal. I sent her a brief email, and she replied right away, indicating that she enjoyed our profile and that she had opened her private photos. Surprised to have been contacted back so quickly by the elusive single female, I foolishly unlocked for her our own private photos, a few of which contain nudes. And, of course, that was the last we heard from her.

My initial deduction from this chain of events was that she'd seen our photos and been unimpressed. Single women, of course, have their pick of pretty much any couple they choose. But then, Tyler gave me "the look", and I realized I'd screwed up. Big time. He had just chatted with a single male friend of ours on the site, they'd compared notes, and after a little bit of digging around, they determined the profile was a complete fake. The certifications turned out to be bogus, from other fake accounts, and the "woman" had changed her city and state on her profile half a dozen times since the day before. This individual was casting a *very* wide net in an attempt to scoop up as many explicit photos as possible from unsuspecting couples. And my dumb self ended up in the net too. I'm now under strict orders to *never* send our private photos to anyone who hasn't proven they are real.

Still, I had to laugh at the irony of shelling out advice about how to avoid picture collectors, as I fell into one's trap that same week.

The moral of the story is that sadly, even "trusted" swinging sites are burdened with their fair share of fake profiles set up for the sole purpose of picture collecting. It's an almost unavoidable reality, and they're clearly getting more and more clever. Here are some experiences couples have shared regarding being tricked by duplicitous photo collectors.

I like to chat on a few swinger websites during the day, it makes my day at the office less boring. One day, a single woman who had just signed up on the site started chatting with me. My wife and I have been looking for a "unicorn" (single female) to hook up with, because that's something we've never had the chance to do. This woman was saying all the right things. Complementing my wife's photos,

telling me I was hot, telling me all the things she would like

to do with us. I should have known something was up, but I

admit, I was getting a little hot and bothered by the

conversation. She was talking about meeting us out that

night, she said she lived near us, had just broken up with

her boyfriend, and wanted to have some dirty fun with a

couple. I was all in! She sent me a face photo through

chat, then she sent me several nude photos which did not

have her face in them. I was surprised that a woman was

so eager to send me nude pics! Then she asked for some x

rated photos of my wife. Not me, just my wife. I thought

that was strange. I remembered some friends telling me

about all the fake people on swinger sites, so I started to

worry. My wife and I had just watched the show Catfish

the night before. The host of the show used an online

image search to look up a photo and see if a person was

real. I immediately put one of the photos she sent me into an image search and it brought up a Facebook page. Of an 18 year old high school student who lived 2,000 miles away and was a member of some big church group. I freaked out and immediately closed the chat. A chat window popped up a few more times, each time asking when I was sending those photos to "her." I haven't chatted online since.

~ Barry, NJ

My husband and I had a "female" of a couple from here out herself as a liar on yahoo chat. While talking to her she just couldn't get her webcam working for SOME reason (yeah right). She sent a few pics. Skip forward a few weeks and we chat with her "husband." He sends a pic of them as a couple. Totally different girl in that pic! Hmmmm... Asking for voice verification may be a good idea that we will try since so many web cams are "broken" when these people chat...

Sara, Fairhope, AL

On more than a few occasions, we have been burned by the infamous "picture collector." They seem to be getting more and more skilled at pretending to be couples interested in meeting. They spend the time to chat with you and make themselves seem real, but as soon as you so much as email a photo of your wife without clothes, the chats and emails stop. There is so much free porn on the internet, I just don't understand why these freaks can't just get it there instead of wasting our time and energy and making us think they are a couple who want to meet us.

~Chad, OK

I feel so stupid. My husband and I discuss all the time about how many fakes are out there when you are looking online to meet people. I look at the Craigslist ads from time to time, mostly for a laugh, but we have actually met a

13

few people from them and it's gone okay. A few weeks ago I noticed a post of a young couple who was coming to town the next night and looking to meet another couple. Everything about the post seemed sincere. They were fairly new to swinging, they asked that people be honest about their age and other stats, since they were being up front about theirs, and they seemed open to all kinds of play despite being new. I emailed them and just sent a face photo. I told my husband I was sure they wouldn't reply. Well, I got a reply five minutes later. She thanked me for the email and told me more about what they were looking for. She said she would send some photos of the two of them. She then sent three emails, each with 8 or 10 pictures. I REALLY should have seen the red flags then and there. But my hope that they were real took over, and I sent them 4 or 5 nude pics of us. We never ever send pics like that unless we have verified people are real. Of course that was the last we heard of them. My husband looked up the photos they'd sent, and all of them were on an amateur

porn site. We're just hoping OUR photos aren't the next to

end up on that site. Lesson learned.

~Suzy, MT

One night we ran into a couple we'd talked to several

times before. As we chit chatted about work, family, and

swinger related stuff, the subject of all the fakes online

came up. My husband began telling him a story about how

he'd busted this pic collector while chatting online. She

couldn't keep her story straight, and he caught onto her

right away. He immediately called her out on being a fake

and she closed the chat window. Well, it turns out this

other couple had been talking to the same woman online

for months. He'd even sent her many photos and video of

his wife, most of which were x rated. He was certain that

this was a real single woman and that if he kept sending

her stuff they would eventually meet. When my husband broke the news to him, he just shrugged and said, "Well, you never know. She may be real after all." He was too excited with the idea of meeting this fake woman to realize that he was sending nude photos and video of his wife to someone who was probably a dude on the other side of the country.

~Annie, Seattle, WA

As you can see, this phenomenon is not rare, and it seems to happen to pretty much everyone at some point. If you are looking to meet people online for dating or sex, you *will* eventually come across a picture collector. So be careful, and look out for the warning signs. Possible hints that someone is a picture collector:

- They claim to be a couple but use the word "I" instead of we whenever talking about "themselves."

- They claim to be a single woman, but they immediately begin chatting in a sexually explicit manner and/or asking for explicit photo or video

- They have a profile on a swingers site, and the profile location keeps jumping to various locations around the country, where each day they are listed as living in a different city.

- They seem more focused on chatting and sharing photos than on making plans to meet. When you ask about meeting, they always have an excuse for not being able to.

- They have a free swingers website profile of a single woman, with a brief written section and a few photos of a thin, attractive, young woman. They usually have no certifications, but lately some smart collectors will make multiple profiles and certify themselves.

If you want to protect yourselves before sending photos and/or agreeing to meet a new couple or single, you might want to take some simple steps to verify that they are who they say they are. You can ask to webchat, as most people these days can do that via pc, smartphone, or iPad. If you'd rather not do a video chat, you can ask them to send you a candid photo from their phone in which they are doing something unique such as touching their finger to their nose, making a hand gesture, or something of that nature. If it's a couple, make sure both members of the couple are in the photo or video. If the photos match what you've already seen on their profile, chances are, they are legitimate. If they make excuses why they can't even send a candid photo, you have reason to believe something isn't right with their story. Either they are picture collectors, or they are otherwise not who they claim to be. Be smart, and that will ensure you have mostly positive experiences with interacting and sharing photos with people online.

Chapter Two

When the Internet and Reality Collide – Badly

Picture collectors are a sad reality when it comes to making connections online. Another more insidious common complaint, however, is that many profiles on swinging sites are less than honest when it comes to details of age, weight, and appearance. We've personally interacted with many couples online, only to run into them while out and discover their photos were at least ten years old, and they were in fact at least 30 pounds heavier than their pictures indicated. While I understand the desire to present your best self in an online profile and when sending photos to prospective new friends, who wants to subject themselves to the disappointed stare of a couple who thought they were meeting a 28 year old size 2, only to encounter a 40 year old size 14? We make a point to always keep updated photos on our own profile; I don't want anyone meeting me and saying, "Damn, you looked better online." How horrifying!

While we've definitely had shocking instances where photos didn't remotely match up with reality when meeting new people, our most perplexing involved a situation where the entire profile simply didn't match a couple we ended up meeting. We noticed a profile of a younger couple who had moved to town recently, and from their photos and profile, they seemed attractive, adventurous, and fun. We emailed and made plans to meet, thinking if things didn't work out in terms of chemistry, we could at least have some fun new friends to go dancing with and otherwise hang out with.

Well, we met this couple about a week after initially emailing them. She did not resemble her photos in more than a cursory way; she was a lot shorter and quite a bit chunkier than her photos let on. We weren't put off by this, though, and we hoped for the best. Within 5 minutes of sitting down with them, we discovered that it's not only photos that can lie; it's also apparently personalities! Gone was the fun, adventurous vibe we'd detected in their profile. This couple was about ten years younger than us, but they acted like they should be on the waiting list for a nursing home.

As we enjoyed beers, they sipped soda, and their conversation involved how much they didn't like living in our city, and how much better their previous home was. We love our city, so this was not the best way to start a potential new friendship. The conversation then turned to religion – they are devout, and we are the furthest from. They seemed openly disturbed by this fact, as we sat there wondering what in the hell we'd gotten ourselves into. They were, to put it generously, dreadfully dull.

We ended the date after about an hour of painful conversation, and we briefly discussed getting together another time. Tyler and I agreed on the way home that we had no interest in meeting with them again, and we talked about how that was *not* the couple we'd expected to meet based on their profile. To be polite, I texted them with a quick thank you for getting together with us. They did not reply. Tyler, not knowing I'd texted them, sent them a similar text the next day. She replied, saying, "We did not feel there was any chemistry and have no interest in further contact." *Ouch!* We were relieved, though, as we would not have seen them again regardless. Hard to have chemistry when one couple barely has a *pulse.* While this story is mild in terms of the outright deception in online profiles, here are some other couples' and singles' experiences with more flagrant dishonesty.

A couple who lived in a neighboring town emailed us

on a swing site and wanted to meet. They had about a

dozen photos of the female, none of the male. And the faces

were blocked out on all of the photos. We felt a little

uncomfortable meeting people when we had never seen

their faces, so we asked them to email us a face photo.

They said they could not, because they were very prominent

in the community. As we examined the photos a bit more,

we realized the backgrounds looked like several different

living rooms. This seemed strange. Then we noticed they

looked sort of like scans of pictures from magazines. The

closer we looked, the more it seemed like it wasn't even the

same woman in each picture. We knew something was up,

so we did not make plans to meet them. A few months later

we ran into them at a swing party. The husband recognized

us and introduced him and his wife. We were floored.

Those photos were not her. She was at least twenty years

older and didn't even have the same body type. She was

also one of the least attractive women we've ever seen. We had no idea what to do. We were thankful that tons of people showed up, and we were able to get away from them. We felt so relieved we never made plans to meet them for drinks. It would have been a very awkward experience.

~ Tricia, Gulfport, MS

My husband had a fantasy of a gang bang, with me as the center of attention. He spent a lot of time emailing and getting pics from people so that he could choose just the right ones. He invited 6 guys to a hotel the night of my birthday; he figured half would show up. Four guys came to the hotel, and only one of them looked anything like his pics. The others were much heavier and older than the pics they sent, and one of them didn't even seem to be the same person. My husband was so angry he sent those three guys

packing. They were pissed. We ended up having a nice
threesome with the one guy who had been honest. We hope
to see him again!

~ Lucy, NV

Shortly after we had started swinging and posted
pictures of ourselves on different sites online, we were
contacted by email by a couple. They sent us our own
photos saying it was them when they contacted us…

~Anonymous

We met a couple for drinks a few years ago, and we
had quite a shock. As with many online profiles of couples,
they had posted 50 or more photos of her, but only one or
two of him, and they were blurry and far away. They kept
making excuses for not being able to update their photos or

send us new ones. She was hot, though, and they seemed

nice, so we agreed to meet. He wanted us to come right

over and get in their hot tub, which freaked us out a little,

so we suggested drinks at a bar near their house. And if

things went well, we could go to their place. When we got

to the bar we recognized her right away. She was in her

early twenties and very cute. We sat next to her, wondering

where her husband was. Then she turned to the OLD man

next to her and introduced him. This man looked nothing

like the blurry photos online. He had salt and pepper grey

hair, a thick mustache, and he looked like he was in his

fifties. Not his thirties as the profile said. We felt totally

creeped out. My wife immediately began fiddling with her

phone as I tried to think of something to say other than oh

my god you're old. She then grabbed my arm and told the

couple there was an emergency at home and we had to go.

Thank goodness for cell phones. It's a shame you can't

leave bad feedback on swinger profiles, like on ebay. Not

as advertised! Would save people the trouble.

~Ed, MD

If you're in the lifestyle, this sort of thing will happen to you at some point. Lately, as mentioned in the previous chapter, we've decided to start asking for candid photos to be texted to us before we agree to meet couples individually. That way, we know for sure they are who they say they are, and that they'll look like we expect. Then again, we're meeting a couple this weekend at a party, and we haven't even seen their faces. Ah, sometimes we never learn!

Chapter Three

The Swinger Stand Up

I've never understood the concept of standing someone up for a date. It's thoughtless and shows a complete lack of common courtesy. It seems that in the world of swinging, standing someone up is even more common than in dating. Part of it most likely stems from the fact that these are mostly "no strings attached" situations, without the potential for feelings or any sort of lasting relationship. Very little is invested in it from the outset, so there's little feeling of regret for blowing someone off. That's an unfortunate reality, and it's completely disrespectful. Even single men, who seem desperate for a couple to even reply to their emails, can become flaky when it comes time to arrange a date with a couple.

Another reason for this discourteous behavior, at least from our own observations and experience, is that couples will often begin to feel a need to weigh all their options until the very last minute. Rather than decide to meet a couple and stick with that decision, they make plans, then continue to send out emails, chat with people, and see if a "better" offer comes along. It's as if they have only that one weekend to have fun, and they don't want to make the wrong decision. A kid in a candy store being told they can have *one* piece of candy, paralyzed with the abundance of choices, certain he'll miss out on finding that perfect piece of candy.

When a couple makes tentative plans for the weekend with us on a Monday, then seems to "disappear" until Saturday, not replying to emails although it's clear they're online, we tend to get a sense that this is what's happening, and by Saturday we've lost all interest. Meanwhile, they've most likely contacted half a dozen couples about meeting, and they're agonizing over which to choose. My hope is usually that *all* the couples will end up blowing them off, and that they'll learn their lesson. Apparently, this sort of thing happens to most swingers, and it's not just restricted to couples.

One thing we hate about trying to meet people in the swinging scene is that they seem to be really wishy washy. The swingers website we use has party listings, and people can sign up on the site to show they are attending the party. Well, to us the nice thing about that is that we can see who will be at the party and if we like someone's profile, we can make plans to meet them at the party and see if there's a connection. We've had good luck with this and met several couples that way. But more often than not, we'll email a couple about meeting for a drink at the party and they will reply saying "we prefer to just play it by ear." Why is it so hard to agree to introduce yourselves and share one drink

31

with people? Or we will have people say "okay, see you there" but then we never end up meeting them because the party is packed. My wife really prefers chatting a bit with people before a party to make a connection, but lately no one seems to want to make the effort to get to know each other. It's too easy to just get drunk and randomly hook up with a total stranger, I suppose. That's not for us.

~Jeff, Macon, GA

This was really embarrassing. I'm a single woman who used to be in the lifestyle. I had a date for dinner and drinks with a couple, and I showed up to the restaurant a few minutes late. I texted them as I was walking to the door to let them know I was there. I walked in and sat at the bar, waiting for a text back. I thought they may be running late too. Then out of the corner of my eye I saw them sitting in the back corner of the restaurant. I was about to get up and walk over to them when my phone vibrated. It was a text from the couple saying they had something come up and couldn't make it to meet me. I was standing at the bar freaking out. The couple obviously saw me and decided to bail on the date. I've never felt so uncomfortable in my life. I sent them a candid photo of me just the day before. I don't know what their problem was, but I guess I didn't live up to their expectations. I think I'm pretty damned hot! So much for single women never getting rejected.

~ Tara, Colorado Springs, CO

I travel a bit for work, and when I'm on the road I sometimes meet up with couples or single women for some fun, with the permission of my wife, of course. One evening when I was spending the night out of town, I got an email from a couple who said they'd like to meet. We exchanged numbers, and they said they'd meet me at a bar near my hotel. I was tired after a long day of work, but I showered, got ready, and went to the hotel. I texted them when I arrived. No reply. I had a drink and sipped it for thirty minutes, not wanting to have too much to drink before meeting them. Still nothing. I texted them to ask if something had come up, but they didn't reply. Thinking they might be driving and not checking their texts, I waited another half hour. By that point I knew they had stood me up. I went back to the hotel and checked my email, just in case. Nothing. I was irritated by the situation, but I know sometimes people can be total jerks, particularly to "single" guys. I pretty much forgot about the whole thing until six months later, when the same couple emailed our couples profile wanting to meet. Before I had a chance to reply, my wife did. And boy, did she tell them off. By the time I got back to my computer, they had blocked us. Idiots.

~Mark, Metairie, LA

One thing that confuses me more than anything in this

"lifestyle" is getting stood up and blown off by single men!

It seems they should be the happiest of anyone to have a

couple take interest in meeting them, but they seem most

likely to be complete jerks and ruin a potentially good

situation. One time, I spent probably two weeks chatting

and emailing this one guy who seemed really nice and

respectful, and he was interested in trying his first

threesome with a couple. Well, the night we were supposed

to meet for drinks, he had to work late. We've been there,

and we totally understood. Then we made plans for a few

days later, and he was "under the weather." Okay, well,

that's cool, we just went out anyway and had a good night

together. We made plans one more time the following

week, and he just didn't reply at all that day to confirm.

We texted and emailed, and got nothing back from him. We

went on with our lives, admittedly a bit peeved at this jerk, and a week or so later he sent some rambling email about how he had been going through a lot, blah blah blah, and that he just wasn't in a good place to meet new people. Whatever.

Fast forward 3 or so years to last month. Again, we decided to try to meet up with a guy. Perused through a bunch of emails in reply to an ad we posted, and we picked the guy who seemed most intelligent and respectful, not some jerk who sent us ten cock photos without bothering to show us his face. Yuck. So my husband texted back and forth with him for a week or so, and we made plans to meet for a drink or two one weeknight. Two days prior, he texted us and said the weather looked bad for that night, did we still want to go? That seemed odd to me. We said yes, we're still on. Then the next day, he sent a strange series of texts about how he just had to juggle too many things, and he was stressed out, and he could meet us, but he would have two friends with him, and would we mind that. Realizing we were dealing with yet another total

flake, my husband just told him to get in touch with us when

his life calmed down. We haven't heard from him since.

For now, we're just going to go to the local club on the

nights single guys are there, and try our luck with that. It's

just not worth all the effort, really.

~Michelle, Allen, TX

We'd had two dates with a really cute, really nice

couple, and while we'd hoped to play with them, the couple

got really shy on the second date and didn't go through

with it. It was no big deal to us, and we kept in touch with

them. They texted us and told us they wanted us to be

"their first" swinging experience, and they couldn't wait to

make it happen. We made plans to get together about a

week and a half later at a party going on in town. 5 days

before, he texted us and said they were sick and wouldn't

be able to make it. We said no problem, but if you feel better, we have 5 more days til the party. He insisted they were just not going to be well enough. We figured they were chickening out of playing and we told them there was no pressure. We didn't hear from them again. We went to the party and saw them walk in with another couple. They looked horrified to see us there and couldn't make eye contact with us. Finally about an hour into the party he came over to try to make small talk. My wife wouldn't even look at him. We have no time for rude people who cancel plans with us and can't even be honest.

~Ernie, Salt Lake City, UT

Sometimes life gets in the way of fun, and we all have had situation in which we've needed to cancel plans we've made with other people. The normal rules of common courtesy should apply in swinging just as in other facets of life, though. Letting people know immediately when plans

must be changed or canceled should be common practice.

Unfortunately, people in general are thoughtless, and

people in the swinging community seem to be burdened

with an extra dose of inconsideration.

Chapter Four

How Rude!

In swinging, just as in life, we all encounter people who simply lack the social skills to function adequately in a group setting. Even worse, we sometimes encounter people who know better, but choose to behave like knuckle-dragging mouthbreathers. I've had a good number of people share with me their stories of such encounters, and I've actually been shocked by the outright sleaziness and rudeness with which some people conduct themselves. That being said, I'll start off with one of our own experiences that didn't make it into my last book. It's amusing, and we still laugh about it.

While some people go to swing clubs hell-bent on meeting people and having sex with someone new each time they attend a party, my husband and I have a different take. We find it to be a lively, enjoyable atmosphere for sharing drinks and laughs with friends, and the different areas of our "home" club afford us the opportunity to laugh and get loud and silly, or to sit in a quieter spot and talk, or, if the mood strikes, to have some sexy fun in one of the many play rooms on the upper floors. We rarely go with the intention of "hooking up" with anyone; sometimes it happens, and we consider that a bonus (if it goes well, that is). Our perspective and behavior in this regard seem to befuddle many of the hardcore swingers who walk into the club and immediately seek out their prey for the night.

One night, we were at the club with four other friends, two of whom we hadn't seen in a while. As I recall, it was a particularly fun night, we all had a little too much to drink, and we spent hours talking, catching up, telling funny stories about recent events, and just having a fantastic time. As we sat and talked, couples entered and exited the room where we all sat. Sometimes they'd sit for a while, and we may or may not have greeted them in some way. There were lulls in the conversation during which time we said hello and introduced ourselves to a few people, but then there were times we were deeply involved in a story and didn't even notice other people coming and going. We must have sat on the comfy upstairs couches for hours, and before we knew it, it was nearly three o'clock in the morning. We hugged everyone goodbye, retrieved our liquor bottle from the bartender, and headed home, thrilled with the fun night we'd had.

The next morning, we hopped online to check our email, and we went to the swingers website we're members of to see what was happening there. We had one email, from a couple who had emailed us a week or so before saying they would like to meet, but had never sent us any face photos of themselves. The email simply said this: "Just wanted to let you know you're not as cool as you think you are." Tyler and I read the email, looked at each other, read the email again, and just sat there, completely puzzled by the cryptic message.

We read the couple's profile, then we looked back at our email history. They were a fairly new couple on the website, and they had indeed emailed us a week or two before, saying they went to the club from time to time and would love to meet us. We'd replied and said that sounded great, but could they send us a picture so we would know who to look for. They never sent a photo. We get quite a few random emails like this, so we didn't give it another thought.

We replied to them, politely informing them that we did not, indeed, fancy ourselves cool by any stretch of the imagination, and inquiring as to why they felt compelled to send us that email. After a series of half a dozen more messaged riddled with grammatical errors and a general lack of understanding of, well, *anything*, it became evident that this couple had wandered into the room in which we were talking to our friends, had sat near the doorway and stared at us, waiting for us to jump up and acknowledge them, and had then left the room in a huff when that acknowledgement did not take place. Still fuming with the pain of rejection, they felt compelled to email us with an insult in an apparent attempt to make themselves feel better.

Once we'd puzzled out what happened, we found the entire thing hilarious. We clued them in to the fact that we were not being rude to them at the club; that we simply had no idea who they were, and that had they come over and said hello we'd have introduced them to everyone and they would have been welcome to join us. They realized it had just been a misunderstanding, and they apologized. Funny thing is, though, that they never did send us a face photo, so for all we know we've sat near them many times since and had no idea it was the couple with which we'd had such a bizarre exchange.

This experience was mild compared to many, but it was an amusing one we always look back on and have to laugh about. We've had more than our fair share of encounters gone awry in more serious ways, but we've been fortunate enough to have not come across many people like those in the following experiences which other swingers have shared with me.

My husband and I hadn't been out in a while, and we knew there was a big party in town for a swingers' convention. We figured that would be a good night to go out, people-watch, and maybe meet some nice couples too. It turned out to be even more packed at the party than we expected, and we sat at the bar, practically unable to move due to the amount of people. Just as I was about to try to get up to look for the restroom, the male half of a couple we'd talked to earlier in the night walked up and stood between us to get a drink at the bar. Before I knew it, he

was leaning up against me, WAY too close, and I was

completely pinned against the bar. He began to rub his

cock against my thigh, through his jeans, and he was

clearly enjoying it. I tried to get my husband's attention,

but he was talking to someone on the other side of him, and

it was so loud he didn't hear me call his name. The

"rubbing" got a little more intense, and I began to literally

feel sick. Finally I jerked the barstool back and shifted my

body so that he couldn't get to me. I really wish I'd

punched him in the face.

~Cara, Reno, NV

My husband and I were contacted after we put up a

post online looking for couples. The couple sent photos to

us, and we sent some to them. They seemed very nice and

very interested in meeting us. The husband gave us his cell number, and we texted back and forth a few times. He

suggested we meet at a bar near the hotel they were staying

at, and then we could go have some fun back in their room.

Sounded good to us! When we met at the bar, his wife

acted very standoffish, almost angry. He played it off and

said she'd lost some money at the casino earlier that day.

We talked a bit, and we probably had too much to drink.

So much that we didn't realize how much she was not into

us, or the situation.

We all kind of stumbled back to their hotel room, and

once we got into their room and sat on the edge of the bed,

she freaked out and pulled him out into the hall. We heard

raised voices, and it went on for some time. We had no

idea what to do. The husband came back in, alone, and

admitted that his wife had no idea he had planned any of

this, he was hoping if he surprised her with it she would

have some drinks and warm up to the idea. We were

horrified. She was nowhere to be seen, and we quickly got

our things and got the hell out of there. Now we always insist on talking to the wife before we agree to meet people we have never met in person before.

~ Cindy, NJ

We had a threesome at a club with a guy we'd spent some time talking to, and my wife found him attractive. I made it clear to him that the ONLY rule was to use a condom. Beyond that, anything goes. He said he totally understood and agreed. What do you know, we get into the room, things start getting hot and heavy, I look down, and there he is, no condom, attempting to fuck my wife. Right in front of me. I ran his ass out of the room, resisting the urge to punch him out. I don't get why guys have to be such idiots.

~Jeff, Macon, GA

We were sitting at the bar of a swing club, and we

witnessed this exchange. The club had just opened for the

night, and there were only a few couples there. A couple

who clearly had been drinking for hours walked in and sat

down next to another couple. The man began to speak to

the couple, and within minutes he was asking the other man

where he worked, and asking him his last name. The man

seemed to not want to say, but the drunk guy pushed the

issue. "Come on, we're all friends here." The couple just

looked really uncomfortable as the guy went on and on,

being very obnoxious and pushy. Then the drunk guy stood

up, no more than 5 minutes later, and asked the other

couple if they wanted to go have sex. The couple looked

stunned and declined. The guy and his wife practically

stormed off. They returned half an hour or so later, asked

AGAIN, and we saw the couple walk off with them. We are

still confused about why that couple went ANYWHERE with those obnoxious people.

~Suzy, Hollywood, FL

My husband and I were sitting in one of the play areas of a sex club, and another couple approached us and began talking to us. The husband was very quiet and reserved, but the wife was super flirty and seemed very interested. After ten minutes or so of chatting, she invited us into one of the small play rooms. We figured what the hell, so we went with them. Once we were in the room, things got a little uncomfortable. The wife was all over me and completely ignoring my husband. When he tried to approach her she literally shoved him away, then she looked at me and said, "I wish it was just the two of us in here." I told her that she had been rude to say that right in front of my husband, and she flipped out on me. She yelled at us and called us "cra-za-zy" as we quickly dressed and left the room. We were so happy they were from out of town, because we really don't want to run into them again.

~Jennifer, Dallas, TX

We'd gotten an email from a couple who saw that we had signed up online for a swingers party happening in our hometown. They were driving in from a few states away just for the party, and they said they wanted to meet and hang out with us that night. We exchanged photos and emails and some texts, and the guy even texted just before the party saying "See you soon!" Well, an hour into the party they showed up, and he came over, introduced himself, and said they'd see us in a little bit. His wife never did even come over and say hello to us. Our photos were all very recent and accurate, so we figured she hadn't even known we existed, it was just the husband emailing, hoping *we could hook up. She apparently wasn't having it. It wasn't cool, though, to be so bitchy about it. Have some decorum and at least be polite! Or don't let your spouse email and make plans with people without consulting you first!*

~ Doug, Birmingham, AL

We met, and hooked up with, a cute couple while out at a club one night. We had a great night laughing and talking, and the sex was great. They contacted us a few months later and we hooked up again, but the second time things just didn't go so great. He was drunk and it just wasn't a good time for me, and my husband also found the situation to be lacking. Now, every time we run into them at that same club, the guy feels like because we've had sex, although it was years ago, he can just walk up to me and

grab my boobs or make really inappropriate comments. I
suppose some would say "anything goes" at a swing club,
but I think some things are just crude and not okay, no
matter what you have done with someone in the past.
Instead of having people we might enjoy having a drink and
catching up with, we see them and want to hide.

~Vanessa, CA

My wife and I attended a meet and greet at a bar. It
was hosted by a website, and we were just looking into this
lifestyle and thought it would be a good chance to meet
other people and find out more about it. Well, don't you
know, as soon as we walked in, I recognized someone from
work. He's kind of an ass, and known to be very rude and
crude around the office. He kept staring at me, but he
didn't come over to talk. I wondered if I should go say
hello, but my wife told me maybe it would just make things

weirder. At the end of the meet and greet, he walked past me, slapped me on the back, and said "See you at the office Monday, Johnny Boy!" Now every time I go to work I'm wondering if our little "secret" has been shared with anyone else. We haven't even done anything in the lifestyle yet, but half the office probably knows we're "swingers." Now I know why some people say they only swing when they go out of town.

~John, OR

We met a guy for drinks one night, when my wife and I first started thinking about trying a threesome. Within thirty seconds of meeting him, we knew it wouldn't go any further. He was nice enough, but he was dumb as rocks and a terrible conversationalist, and after an hour we told him we needed to head home. He texted us that night and asked when we were going to get together again. We said we didn't think it would work out. He continued texting

every day for two weeks, with everything from "your wife is

hot" to "really want to meet up again" to "come on, man,

let's get together." I never replied after the first text. It's

no wonder some of these guys are single and desperate for

sex. They have NO social skills at all. We are glad we

knew right away we wanted nothing more to do with this

guy – because he sure did turn out to be a weirdo.

~Alan, Boise, ID

My boyfriend and I replied to a post on Craigslist. It was a

couple looking to have fun with another couple. We're pretty

experienced with swinging, but we had not had any fun like that

in a while. We texted back and forth with the couple; they sent

us both their cell numbers and my boyfriend and I sent several

messages and exchanged photos. They both seemed decent

looking and like they were serious about meeting. We agreed to

meet them at a bar across town. We showed up, and we

recognized the guy right away. He was sitting alone at the bar,
so we thought his wife was in the restroom. We introduced
ourselves, and he seemed very nervous. We asked about his
wife, and he said she was still at the hotel, that she had a
headache and would be walking over soon. We thought that was
really weird, but we decided to wait. We had some beers and
talked to him, and he seemed very reserved compared to his
texts. He was nice enough, though, so we figured we'd give it a
chance. He kept checking his phone, and he finally said she was
feeling better and we could go meet at the hotel. I felt something
was really off, so I excused myself and texted her from the
restroom. There was no reply. When I went back to the bar and
told him I'd texted her and not heard back from her yet, he
practically turned white as a sheet. He fiddled with his phone
again, then said he needed to go, and he rushed out without even
really saying goodbye. We're still not sure what was waiting for
us at the hotel, but we're certain it wasn't a wife.

~ Sandy, Chicago, IL

I had hit up a couple on SLS a long time ago, and was given the response of, "Thanks for your interest, but if and when we're interested in a single guy, we'll contact you." Not uncommon, lots of couples feel that way, and since they didn't have "NO MEN NO MEN NO MEN" plastered all over their profile, I decided to say "hello."

About 3 weeks ago, I received another message from them saying that they would be vacationing in the area, and wanted to know if I could come over for an evening of play. I told them that I was definitely still interested, and that all I needed was a time and place. After 2-3 weeks of the wife and I talking back and forth, and her telling me how hot she was getting by the thought of us finally meeting, I was pretty stoked to meet these people also. She had asked for a cock pic, now I don't have XXX rated pics on my page...because most ladies would like to see a nice shot of the face and body in a PG setting first and foremost. I gladly will send one on request though. I did send her one, granted the angle makes it look huge, but I told her that it was 6"...so as not to "false advertise" myself. She said that it looked great, and that she would enjoy playing with it.

I arrived to the hotel and they seemed like very nice people, he and I chatted quite a bit and began teasing her with some dumb jokes. Things started heating up, and some oral was exchanged between her and I and eventually he joined in. After maybe 30 minutes, she began complaining of heartburn. We stopped and began to just chat to see if maybe she would feel better. While we were chatting, we talked about our experience in the lifestyle and what got us here and so forth. I had told them that I love being in a close-knit group of people where I feel like there is so much trust. However, the lifestyle contains 2 polar types of people...the best of the best, and the worst of the worst. I love that I've met so many people that I can trust and become really close friends with. They are almost like a family, and there are things that I can go to them with in confidence that I wouldn't even tell blood relatives.

But...unfortunately, there are people who just have no

manners, are shady, flaky, or just fake about who they are.

They agreed completely, and I told them that even

though she felt sick, I was very glad to have met them, they

seemed like amazing people, and that I would love to stay

in touch. They said the same, noting that she was attracted

to me and that he and I got along very well. She had been

apologizing about being sick ever since it happened, to

which I said that it wasn't her fault. Things like that

happen, and I wasn't upset in the least. I thanked them,

hoped that she was feeling better soon, and left.

The next morning I jumped on-line to check all of my

messages of sorts...when I got to SLS, I noticed that they

had written me. Expecting another apology about her being

sick, I opened their message to find something to the effect

of. "While we enjoyed meeting you, we felt no connection

between us, and that our profile indicates that she prefers

well endowed men. Good luck in your future swinging

endeavors." I was outraged. The fact that this girl had seen

a picture of my cock and was given the full description of it,

and then had the audacity to call me "small" was just

unbelievable. If she had doubts, she should have either

asked for another photo, or told me up front that she was

no longer interested in meeting. Not to mention the part

about having "no connection," when she even told us that

he and I would get along very well. Now understanding

why she was "sick" made me even more irate, and I told

them that if she wasn't happy with what she saw after I took

my clothes off, she should have said so, and politely asked

me to leave. That would have been much less of a slap in

the face, and saved me 2 hours of my time. I also went on to

say that she should screen her future play partners more

carefully to avoid similar situations and wasting others'

time as well as your own...I was professional in that I didn't curse them out or anything, but let them know that I was

very displeased with their decision on handling the whole

thing. Of course, I was promptly blocked from their profile

and messages afterwards...

People like this are the reason why others have doubts,

or begin to have doubts about the lifestyle. I was very

insulted, not because she wasn't happy with my dick

size...but in the way that she wasted my time and essentially

lied when she said that it looked "Good enough for her." I

feel bad for anyone else who decides to get to know them

further. They're 2 faced and very immature. This is the 2nd

worst experience that I've ever had...

~Ben, Tampa, FL

Admittedly, swinging, and the interactions it entails, is
not remotely the "norm" of social interaction in society.

There are different rules of etiquette with swinging than with, say, interacting with other couples at an employee picnic (to say the least). There *are,* however, rules of etiquette, and people who don't realize that they should still behave like civilized, kind human beings have no place in the swinging world.

Unfortunately, swinging also tends to attract some individuals and couples who are using swinging as a "quick fix" for problems they have in their lives. Single men who can't find or keep a girlfriend might turn to hooking up with couples for the sexual release they can't find through dating. But if they can't behave in such a manner to hang onto a girlfriend, they likely can't handle the social intricacies of a threesome either. Similarly, couples might try swinging in a misguided attempt to work out problems in their relationship. Even worse, some individuals in couples try to trick, or coerce, their partner into swinging against their will. This is a recipe for disaster no matter what the details are, and it's downright unacceptable to involve unwitting couples in that sort of duplicity and drama.

Chapter Five

Parties Gone Wild...ly WRONG

While many swingers choose to keep things more intimate, meeting up with couples or singles for a quiet dinner or drinks, or inviting them to their home or hotel, a good bit of swinger socializing takes places at parties and swing club events. While this can be an exhilarating experience, it also opens a couple up to some unexpected scenarios with unanticipated twists and turns. Sometimes those are great and add to the fun, but sometimes it's just all kinds of wrong.

I shared a story of Tyler and me unwittingly going into the group sex room of our local club when no one else was in there at the time. We stupidly thought it would be a good spot for a quickie, and we soon learned that in that room, "anything goes", and in a matter of minutes anything indeed went – and we got the hell out of there after some nonconsensual foot play and a random cock finding its way to my mouth. Well, this is still our favorite club, and we still have fun there, everywhere but the dreaded group room. We were alone in one of the other rooms one night during a crowded party, and in that room, it's understood that no one is to touch you unless invited. It's still a very "open" room, though, but that is sometimes part of the fun.

Tyler and I were naked in the large bed having sex, and we were aware that anyone might hop in the bed alongside us, but in the past when that happened, there was little or no interaction if we didn't know the people. Well, this time, a couple got into bed right next to us, and it was the couple from the group room many months before. My immediate instinct was to jump up and run out the door, but knowing the rules of this particular room, I decided to ignore them. And I did…until a cold hand slowly made its way onto my breast and *squeezed.* We felt them scoot even closer to us, to the point that the man was sweating on us. That, combined with my previous unsolicited experience with them, was more than I could bear. We jumped up in unison, grabbed our clothes and shoes, and walked out, naked, into the hallway to find a more private spot away from that couple.

For a long while, that particular couple seemed to be at the club every single time we showed up, and we were always a bit bummed when we saw them sitting at the bar. We tended to avoid the more public play areas because they made me *that* uncomfortable, and they just didn't seem to have any boundaries based on our own experiences and what we witnessed in their interactions with others. They seemed to lock onto new couples and follow them around, hoping the couple would break down and give in to their advances. Fortunately, we haven't seen them in ages. And we've had more fun because of it!

Unfortunately, swing parties can go much, *much* worse than that, as evidenced by the experiences which others have shared.

We went to our first swinger party in August of 2011. We were in the public play room and in the process of doing a soft-swap (oral only) with another couple, when all of the sudden we hear a man yelling, "Get off of my wife, you bastard!" All four of us freaked out a little bit, unsure of what was happening. The yelling man punched a guy I hadn't noticed yet, standing to our left, and a fight broke out. I ran, naked, into the dancing room, trying to find the host or even some men to break it up. The guys in there just started checking out my naked body, in spite of me telling them that there was a fight in the public room. Finally, a few of them broke up the fight. Both of the fighters had broken and bloodied noses; they got kicked out. Our evening ruined; my boyfriend and I put our clothes back on. Word got out around the party and many other couples came up to us, reassuring us that this usually never happens, and that they hope to see us again at another party. What they said was true...I never witnessed anything like that again.

~ PF, Fresno, California

My boyfriend and I were at the club playing in the group play room. One of the other couples was interested in a full swap with us. We started out, as usual, with girl play. However, the other woman was very drunk and kept giving me sharp little bites all over my body. Now, I like biting (both giving and receiving) but this woman had no idea how to bite properly, so I told her to stop biting me. She didn't, in spite of me telling her about three times. So I told her husband to make her stop biting me. She listened to him; I, however, didn't really want any further contact with her. So we went into a full swap. I was in doggy, so her husband came up behind me; I reached around and felt his cock with my hand, to make sure he was wearing a condom. He wasn't. I sat down on my butt and told him to put on a condom (which he did). I went back into doggy and he penetrated me. At some point, my vaginal juices dried up and sex was beginning to be painful (especially with the condom--too much friction!). When this happens to me, I usually hock up a big wad of spit, put it on my hand, and lube myself up while still fucking the guy. I tried to do so in this situation, but the guy pinned my hands down below me and prevented me from doing so (perhaps he thought I was trying to touch my clit; some men see this as an ego-killer. I try to stay away from those type of men). It was VERY painful after that; I felt like I was being rubbed raw and started making noises of pain instead of pleasure. Finally, he came. In hindsight, I should have known that he would try to be a Dominant ass; he was wearing a leather

cock ring, which is not typical attire for your average

swinger.

~PF, Fresno, California

My husband and I were having sex in the voyeur room

of a club in a city we were visiting for our anniversary. We

found it exciting to be watched, and we had been told that

no one could join us unless they were invited. We were

fucking like mad and quite a crowd was gathering, and the

onlookers made it very exciting. The club where we live

doesn't have a room like this, so we were really enjoying

ourselves. I guess someone else was enjoying it too,

because the husband in one of the couples kept getting

closer and closer until he was practically jerking off in my

face. I was afraid he was going to cum all over me, he was that close. We tried to scoot closer, but he just kept

walking towards us. His wife was sitting against the wall

doing nothing. We ended up grabbing our clothes and

running from the room, leaving a bunch of voyeurs looking

at an empty bed and a masturbating man.

~Katy, Seattle, WA

My wife and I were invited to a hotel party – the

organizers claimed it was a new party and was going to be

one of the most "exclusive" swing parties in town. It was

in a hotel suite downtown, and the cost was only $50 –

cheap for our area. They said everyone who attended had

to be "on the list" so that only the best couples would be in

attendance. I asked about whether singles were allowed,

because my wife gets uncomfortable around a lot of single

guys. They told me that "very select" single men and

women would be invited, but they told me not to worry.

Well, the night of the party arrived, and we decided to give it a shot. My wife spent lots of time getting ready, because we felt we needed to look really nice to fit in with this exclusive bunch of people. When we arrived at the party, we walked in and saw that other than the host couple, it was a room full of men. Must have been a dozen of them crammed into the hotel suite. They looked like zombies wanting some brains when my wife walked in. I was about to ask the hosts when the other couples would arrive, but my wife looked panic stricken. I put my $50 back in my wallet and we went straight back home.

~ Alan, Longmont, CO

We got an email from a couple we met when we attended a Baltimore party saying they were having a party and they even hired entertainment for the party. That entertainment ending up being a very attractive woman putting on a sex show with her black lab. With many of the

guests, it didn't go over very well.

~Sean, RI

We went to our first party for my 31st birthday and we

show up to this two room hotel suite and no lie there was 5

girls and there were at least 20 guys. The other girls there

did not interact much and at midnight they left, explaining

they were only eye candy! Well we stayed hoping the other

ladies were late and we had drove 1 1/2 hours. Well one

other girl showed up wearing only a fishnet bodysuit and

rainbow socks and kept sitting in my lap! I would move and

she would hop back on. I have no problem with women but

I like to be asked before I am touched. Well a couple

started having sex on the floor I front of the TV (the news

was on) and the female who was on top was making idle

chatter with the people in the room. My hubby and I left

quietly. Horrid night, the party had a great reputation too.

~Angel, VA

My wife and I went to New Orleans for our

anniversary, and we decided to try out one of the swingers

clubs in town. One of them was newer, so we thought we

would go there. They were also having a new members

meet and greet weekend, and the price was great!

Unfortunately, the crowd was not so great. After some

uncomfortable exchanges with a few couples, I convinced

my wife to go explore some of the playrooms upstairs, even

if we just had fun together and didn't invite anyone else to

join. Well, on our way up the stairs we passed a shirtless

man who appeared very much "out of it." We didn't know

if he was drunk or on drugs or what. I turned after we

passed him, and his back was covered in blood. I don't

mean a scratch here and there. I mean fresh, wet blood covering his back. We knew there was a BDSM room in the club, as we saw it on our tour. We didn't know anything that intense went on there, and we also didn't think it was appropriate for someone to be walking around a swingers club covered in blood. My wife and I stopped and looked at each other, and we didn't have to say anything. We hightailed it out of there.

~Richard, Little Rock, AR

As a single guy in the lifestyle, I'm often not allowed to attend swing club events or parties; they tend to specify couples and single women only. I got an email recently from a couple on SLS who said they wanted to get together. After a few emails back and forth, they said they were hosting a "small hotel party" and that while they normally didn't invite single men, I was welcome to join them. Oh, *and the cost was $150. They wouldn't tell me anything*

about the party other than that it was in a "nice hotel

room" and that they would provide "finger foods." I asked

about other couples who were attending, and they refused

to tell me any of that. They also had no interest in meeting

me at a bar for a drink before the party. I decided they

were just trying to make some easy cash off of me, so I

declined. They blocked me on SLS after that. I guess they

are only looking for suckers, not for actual friends to have

fun with.

~Tony, NJ

These stories might be enough to scare any semi-sane person away from the mere *thought* of attending a swing party or club event. Fortunately, the majority of parties and events are legitimate, and are populated by couples and individuals who are decent, intelligent, socially aware people. And then when those few odd, even horrifying, things take place, it simply adds to the entertainment of the night. As long as it doesn't happen to *you*!

If there's anything to take away from this chapter, it's the importance of doing your research before attending a party or event. Look for others who have attended or who are members and email them. Ask about the club, the members, and the rules. If it's a hotel party, be *very* wary unless it has a longstanding reputation. Many times, it's just a couple or single person trying to make some quick cash, and their priority is *not* ensuring that the guests have a good time. If you're new to the swinging world, I highly recommend you stick with legitimate clubs; you will be much better off than trying your luck with a random group at a hotel suite.

Chapter Six

Alcohol and the Dumbass Swinger

If you have read my book, *Swinging by a Thread: The Misadventures of an Accidental Swinger*, you know I've had my fair share of experiences with swingers who have had too much to drink. One ended particularly traumatically, and I almost hesitated to include it because it was so awful. But I did, and it seems I'm not the only one who has been the victim of drunk swinging gone horribly wrong.

Another, quite different experience involving the overindulgence of alcohol, happened to us several years ago. We were at our local club, and it was quite a busy night there. We met a guy and his "friend with benefits" who were visiting town for the night. I was quite taken with him almost immediately, which to put it mildly, is *very* rare. Tyler took note of this fact and seemed quite intrigued. Unfortunately, Tyler was nowhere near smitten with the guy's female friend. She was loud, her laugh was something out of a nightmare, and she was generally just a pretty obnoxious person.

We all continued drinking and talking until well past midnight, and at some point the guy and I began kissing. It was lovely, and I admit, I selfishly wanted more despite the fact that that meant encouraging Tyler to give Ms. Obnoxious a chance. He shrugged and said what the hell, so we made our way upstairs. Just before we all piled into one of the small semi-private rooms, she drunkenly looked at Tyler and loudly said, "Wait, *who are you?*" It became clear she was beyond black-out drunk, and I realized we needed to call the whole thing off. We said our goodbyes and headed home. I felt awful for almost getting Tyler into a potentially uncomfortable situation, not to mention the possibility of having sex with someone who was clearly too drunk to consent.

Another night, we'd gone to out drinking and dancing with some friends of ours, and the plan was to go back to their place for some fun. I'd been the designated driver that night, so everyone else really lived it up. When we got back to their house, Tyler, the guy, and I all headed to the bedroom while his wife was busy returning a phone call in the other room. The guy grabbed me roughly and kissed me, then pushed me back onto the bed. He pulled my panties down, slipped two fingers inside me without any warning, then promptly passed out on top of me.

I glanced over at Tyler, who became aware that I had 200 pounds of dead weight on me. He helped push the guy off of me, I got my panties back on, and we decided it was time to head home. It could have been a fun night, but a little too much vodka can spoil the fun for everyone.

I've received more stories than I even have room to include that focus on the hazards of drunk swinging. This first story, however, takes the cake, and the worst part is, I'm sure there are others who have gone through similarly horrifying situation due to overindulgence of alcohol or other substances. The remaining experiences detailed in this chapter are much more common, so much so that I found myself nodding along with each one, remembering my own similar experiences and observations.

Here is MY story. Meet a couple online, do the meet and greet thing at a restaurant. All is good. They invite us to their house the next day. We arrive and they are drunk. She was very very drunk and asked my husband if he wanted to bathe her?!?! He's horny enough to say okay and I'm left with a naked stranger who can barely stand, let alone get an erection. We make out a little bit and my husband comes in the room with the naked, and clean, lady. She proceeds to give him a blow job and her husband falls asleep next to me. I'm very voyeuristic so I watch and she is awful. He grimaces and flinches and eventually FAKES an orgasm. She comes up for air exclaiming how he came a lot. I'm trying not to laugh which gets easy as the smell hits me. She had thrown up on his cock and thought it was cum...I can't get out of there fast enough. Shudder.

~ e. Walker, San Diego, CA

This is unfortunately not the only time something like this happened to us, but it was the funniest. My wife and I were out with a couple we'd been spending time with, and we were drinking and talking and flirting. At one point in the night they suggested we go back to our place for some fun. It was a twenty minute drive, and I figured that might be good, to give the guy some time to sober up. My wife had been the unfortunate recipient of several drunken, limp dicks in the past, and I didn't want that to happen again, especially with a couple we'd really become friends with. Well, to my horror, the guy had a bottle of wine with him, and even though I mentioned to him he should stop drinking, he downed the entire rest of the bottle on the ride to our house. By the time we got home, he was blitzed. He was talking a good game, pulling my wife's hair, acting all manly, even giving her a little slap a few times. But when it came down to fucking her, he couldn't get it up. Instead of getting mad, she just laughed it off and joined us while he sat there trying in vain to get it up. The worst thing is, we gave things another try with them and the same thing happened. After that he knew better than to bother. We stayed friends, though, and he was a good sport about the whole thing.

~James, Pensacola, FL

Some friends joined us in the group sex room of a swingers club, and a hot couple we'd met at the bar earlier asked if they could join. They were both pretty tipsy, but that's not unusual in the club scene. We all had a really good time, and things seemed to be going really well. Then suddenly we heard her yelling for someone to get her a trash can. My friend jumped up and ran, naked, into the hallway to get a trash can for her. He was just in time. She leaned over the side of the bed and threw up for what seemed like hours. We were all in bed, naked, and the mood was so ruined, but no one wanted to be the first one to just get up and get dressed and walk out. So we just kind of lay there, smiling at each other nervously and trying to wait for her to get up and go to the bathroom. She finally did, and by that point we were very happy to all quickly find our clothes and put an end to that part of the night.

~Anthony, Pittsburgh, PN

My husband and I go several times a month to a very

upscale swing club about thirty minutes from our home.

We really like the atmosphere there, and we feel we tend to

meet a higher caliber of people there than at some of the

other clubs and events near our city. One night, though,

the upscale environment was somewhat disrupted. We

arrived at the club very soon after they opened, and there

was only one other couple there. They were at the bar

drinking, and when we said hello to them the wife looked

up and we honestly wondered how she was upright. She

had apparently been drinking for hours. Her eyes were

practically rolling back in her head as she slurred a hello

back at us. We got some drinks and made our way to

another part of the club. About half an hour later, I went to

the restroom. When I opened the door, I saw LEGS coming

out from one of the stalls. The woman was passed out on

the floor, with her face on the tile next to the toilet and her legs extending all the way out of the stall next to the sink.

It wasn't even ten o'clock! I walked out and found an

attendant in the hall – her husband was nowhere to be

seen. I informed her there was a woman passed out in the

restroom, and she contacted the manager immediately. I

walked back to find my husband, and by the time we walked

back the woman was gone. I hope her husband didn't have

to carry her too far to their car or hotel. I just can't

believe anyone would get that drunk that early in the night,

especially when paying nearly $100 to go to a party.

~Christine, LA

We went on a swingers cruise, which to be honest had

all sorts of crazy stories we could tell. But one thing that

we kept noticing which we couldn't get over was this one

older couple. The wife seemed to be drunk from the time

she boarded the ship until the morning we got back to the

port. She looked completely out of it most of the time, and on at least three nights we saw her husband practically dragging her down the halls of the ship to get her to their room. It couldn't have been much fun for him, and she probably doesn't even remember being on the ship. I'm sure this isn't just a thing you see with swingers, but it was definitely a weird thing to see.

~Robert, Montgomery, TX

We have a story about swinging and drinking. Drinking way too much. We were at a party one night, and the entire crowd was drinking freely – however, one woman seemed to take it to a whole new level. After downing more tequila shots than I could handle without being sent to the ER, she decided the thing to do was put on a show on the stripper pole. Well, I just knew this would not end well. A big crowd gathered to watch and cheer her on, and she began to spin around the pole. She tried to climb it a few times, but each time she slid back down. Towards the end of her "routine" she began to get a little too over confident of her skills and her sobriety, and she attempted an upside-down spinning maneuver. She ended up crashing down, head first, onto the stage, and for a minute she just lay there with her head tilted at a horrible angle. No one moved – I think we all thought she broke her neck. Finally her husband came running forward, drink in hand, and pulled her off the stage and onto the nearby sofa. She probably needed a bottle of water, but her idiot husband fed her the rest of his cocktail instead. We didn't stick around to see if she got back on that pole!

~Barry, Chicago, IL

Drinking and swinging seem to go hand in hand, and that's not always a bad thing, particularly when one needs a little liquid courage in order to break the ice. Hell, I hardly remember our first swinging experience because I had downed Long Island Iced Teas like they were going out of style due to my own extreme case of nerves. I've learned, though, that while a drink to kick off the night is a great thing, it's best to drink in moderation, and to choose the company of others who do the same. Too many things can go awry when you have a room full of blizted swingers!

Chapter Seven

Swinging with a Side of Drama

If drinking is common among swingers, then drama is a full-on epidemic. Every profile on a swingers site or post on a hookup site is quick to declare "No Drama!" Well, at least half of the time, that is an outright lie. I have never in my life witnessed as much drama as I've witnessed among people in the swing lifestyle. We've learned, for the most part, how to avoid it, but it was a long and treacherous journey to get to that point. There are couples who are bogged down with jealousy and body image issues, there are couples trying to fix broken relationships, and there are couples who just can't seem to get their acts together long enough to hang out one night without fighting. It's painful enough just spending time with such people, but try getting naked with them and watch the drama amplify to a dangerous volume. Or, better yet, learn from the experiences in this chapter, and stay away from the drama queens!

We've been embroiled in some major craziness throughout our swinging experiences, but there was one amusing bit of drama which we simply bore witness to recently, and which made us thankful we've remained relatively drama-free for a good while now. We were hanging out with five or six couples at a swing club, and some of the group were watching two couples having sex in a windowed room off the main hallway. One of the couples sitting near the window was watching the action rather intently.

The wife in that couple had been telling us of their swinging experiences, and it was quite obvious that they were swinging simply so she could be with other women, and that her husband really wasn't getting much out of it.

This is another dynamic we've learned to steer clear of when meeting people, because it always seems fraught with issues. We were both wondering why they didn't just have an agreement that she could play on her own, because he seemed, frankly, rather bored with the whole thing.

The wife began to ogle the two women in the bed behind the window, and at that point one of the men from the room came out to the hallway. She mentioned how hot his wife was, and he replied, "Well, you're welcome to join us." She practically leapt out of her seat, looking like a kid on Christmas morning, and her husband grabbed her arm. "What are you doing?" he asked her rather sharply. She stumbled over her words, seeming suddenly very nervous. "I didn't say you could go in there," he said to her, still holding onto her arm. "We can just take our asses right home, how about *that?*" And with that, he yanked her down the hallway and they were gone.

The next day, the wife emailed us as though nothing odd had happened. She seemed to think perhaps we'd want to get together with them sometime in the future. No, thank you! Some other couples weren't so lucky, and they found themselves caught up a bit more intimately in other people's drama.

We had a foursome with a couple several years ago, and while they were nice people, we were new to swinging and really wanted to see what else was out there. We didn't want to limit our options. When we didn't agree to hook up with them the next time they asked, they stopped emailing us for a while. We thought nothing of it, as we were busy with life and with meeting new people. We ended up crossing paths again randomly at a party, and we all ended up having sex. They invited us to their house the next weekend, and we met up with them again. Then we got busy with life and family obligations, and we didn't contact them for a month or so. They sent us a hateful email and called us out for being mean and insensitive to them, and they said clearly we weren't "their kind of people", and then they blocked us from emailing them. We had actually intended to get in touch with them again, but were too busy to even think about going out. Apparently they took it WAY too personally and had a complete hissy fit. We have no time for that kind of thing in our lives. When they see us out now, they just ignore us and look the other way. So weird.

~Stacey, NY

We were having sex with a couple we'd met once before and had a lot of fun hanging out with. Everything seemed cool and we thought it would be a good night. In the middle of things, the wife began to look flat out angry. I don't know if she thought her husband was too into my wife, or what. She then grabbed his arm and pulled him over and said "Remember what we talked about! Don't you do it!" My wife and I had no idea what was happening. Then right there, with all of us naked in a bed together, they began to have a debate about why it was okay for him to put his dick in someone's mouth, but not their pussy. Talk about a mood killer. As they continued to argue, we got dressed and waved goodbye and went out to look for some other people with less issues. Fortunately we ran into some other friends and had some fun with no one fighting about it.

~John, Sacramento, CA

The first night we went to this new club (we'd just moved to town) a nice looking couple immediately started hitting on us pretty hard. We'd been drinking at dinner and were feeling no pain, and we went with it and had some fun with them. Well, they seem to think now that

every time we all happen to be at that club together, we

"belong" to them. They practically demand we sit next to

them at the bar, and if we go talk to other people, or god

forbid flirt, they give us major attitude. The other day we

were talking to a single man at the other end of the bar,

and the couple started sending drinks over to us and

waving at us. We knew they were there, we just wanted to

say hello to a friend of ours! I hate to say this, but we keep

hoping they will move away or break up or something,

because they ruin our night when we go out. And they are

always there. I think they must have a room they rent out

in the building. Ha!

~Gina, AZ

We went to a meet and greet at a bar a few months

back. Everyone seemed to already know each other, so we

just sat and looked around. A couple came up and
introduced themselves. They were cute and we thought
they seemed fun. Then they told us how they were both
going through ugly divorces from their spouses, and how
they had started dating a few weeks ago. Within ten
minutes we heard about their custody battles and how her
husband had cheated and about how she was going to take
the house from him. Then the couple asked if we wanted to
go to their hotel room. None of that stuff was our business,
but after hearing all of it we just thought it best to not get
involved with them. Seemed like a lot of mess to get in the
middle of.

~Anthony, IL

I began chatting online with a single guy who was
moving to our city in about a month. We chatted once or
twice a week for that month, and finally he was in town.

He had said he hoped he could get together with me and my husband as soon as he was settled in and finished unpacking. We were excited to meet him, as this was going to be our first MFM threesome. After he'd gotten all moved in, he emailed us about meeting. In the email he said that he had just met a girl before moving, and that they were dating (although it was a long-distance relationship) so we could hang out, but sex was off the table. He was new to the area and had no friends, and still wanted to meet up with us because of that. To be honest, we have enough friends – we were looking for someone we could hook up with.

I told him we weren't able to get together that night. A few days later, since that opportunity was gone, I put up a post online, on another site, for single guys to contact us. The first email I got was from HIM. Saying he was new to town and really wanted to meet a couple to have some threesome fun with. We didn't have a photo posted, so of course he had no idea it was us he was emailing. I was

floored. I replied to his email pretty much saying well,

what happened to your girlfriend? He said he thought

about it and decided it made no sense to be monogamous

with someone he just met and didn't even live in the same

state as. Of course he hadn't bothered to email me before

and tell me he had a change of heart. I don't know what his

deal was, but he seemed to have some major issues and we

never talked to him again after that.

~Ashley, Albany, NY

There's a couple who shows up at a lot of parties we

go to, and it seems every time they are out together they

end up arguing in the corner, then leaving. We sometimes

place bets on how long it will take for them to find a corner

to argue in. I don't know what they fight about, and if they argue all the time at home too. But I think they need to work out their issues before they go to any more parties.

~Sarah, Memphis, TN

My husband and I met a couple online, and we were all interested in meeting. They lived an hour away, so it was going to take a few weeks to arrange a date for the four of us. In the meantime we chatted and texted to get to know them a little bit before meeting in person. Well, the husband started texting me with some sexy messages, complimenting my figure and talking about one of the outfits I had on in some of my photos online. I had no problem with this, I thought it was nice. Then he started texting more explicit things, talking about sex and what he liked and what he hoped to do with me when we met. I went along with it, it was kind of hot and I figured my husband was texting the same sort of things to his wife. We have no

100

problem with this type of flirting and texting with other

people.

Apparently his wife had a big problem, though. I got a
very angry text which was about 6 texts in a row from her
one morning when she must have decided to go through her
husband's phone. She was furious about the sexy texts we'd
sent to each other and she basically accused him of
cheating on her with me. We were all planning to have sex,
so I figured the texting was not a problem. But it was a big
problem for her and she told me to never text or email
either of them again. Of course we never ended up meeting.
That's probably for the best.

~Janet, WA

Drama can rear its ugly head in any social situation,
but when you bring sex into the mix, the potential for
things to get weird rises exponentially. Fortunately, there

are people out there who *do* have their acts together. Of course they may go through periods of trouble, like all relationships, but they strive to keep it between the two of them and not drag others into it. When perusing the swing sites, a common thing to see on a profile is "taking a break." It's good for couples to take a step away from "the lifestyle" now and again, whether they are having issues they need to deal with, or even just to reconnect and spend quality time together, without the distractions of other people.

Chapter Eight

A Swing and a Miss

There are nights we go out, either to meet new people or to see existing friends, and things end up going so bizarrely awry that all we can do is shake our heads in disbelief. These are the times we look back on and just have to laugh, because we simply don't know what else to do. In fact, we had such a perplexing encounter last year that it actually served as the inspiration for me to begin collecting other swingers' experiences for this book. I'd known for a long while that truth is stranger than fiction, but this experience left me and my husband shaking our heads and laughing for months.

Couples new to swinging seem drawn to us. It's a blessing and a curse. A year or so ago, another new couple sent us an email and wanted to meet. They had not had any experiences or met anyone else yet, but they seemed quite certain we were "the" couple they wanted to have their first experience with. We made plans to meet at their favorite bar, and both Tyler and I were really looking forward to it. They seemed like an attractive, genuine couple with whom we thought we could make a nice connection.

We had a quick dinner and made our way to the bar. We'd had a very stressful afternoon, and we were ready to have some drinks and enjoy getting to know our new friends. We found the bar and looked in, seeing only one table near the back occupied by four people. We looked again, and we realized two of the people at the table were the couple we were there to meet. Tyler and I looked at each other, a bit confused by the fact that there was another couple there with them. We thought perhaps they were out with friends, so we made our way to the back of the bar to say hello. The wife jumped up and hugged us hello, then introduced us to her husband, her *daughter,* and her *son in law.* We thought we had seen it all in the wacky world of swinging, but we were downright floored. Stunned and speechless as well, we stood there not knowing quite what to say or do.

The wife began to chat with us and tell us about how they'd talked for quite some time and decided to try swinging. Meanwhile, the son in law literally *leered* at me. He was twenty years younger than me, and it felt like having one of my kids' friends there looking me up and down as I tried to meet a new couple. I don't mind feeling dirty, but I have my limits! I don't think I have ever felt so confused and shocked in my life. I downed a drink in record time as I sat there, nodding along as she talked, and wondering just how in the hell this couple had decided it was appropriate to bring their daughter along on a swing date, and that it was also appropriate to not give us a heads up about it.

After what seemed like hours of horrendously awkward chatting, they mentioned walking up the street to a dance club. I thought that perhaps they'd realized the error of their ways and were going to ditch the kids so we could actually talk and get to know each other. While I wasn't exactly into it, I was glad they'd come to their senses, albeit a little too late. Then I heard the rest of the invitation; the daughter and son in law were accompanying them too. Tyler and I looked at each other, imagining the six of us at a dance club, and to this day I don't know how we both didn't just crack up right in front of the four of them.

I told them it had been a long day, and that we were going to head home. They texted us before we made it to the car, and they expressed an interest in getting together with us again. Tyler texted what was probably the rudest text he's ever sent anyone: "Thanks, but we'll pass." We literally had no other words at that moment. I think our jaws were on the floorboard of the car the entire drive home. We noticed their profile disappeared a few weeks later. Definitely for the best, both for them and for everyone else on the site.

We actually had another completely bizarre experience just this past weekend. I do believe we must be a magnet for weirdoes at this point, because it seems we can't go out without something completely off the wall befalling us. Thankfully, we're much more prone to laugh about it now than we were years ago.

We were out at the swing club, and we'd just gone through week two in a row of meeting a couple we'd had plans with, only to have her get drunk and pass out by midnight, ruining any chance of having a fun night together. We shrugged it off and decided to talk to some new people who were at the club for the first time. After an hour or so of jovial chatting, not to mention sharing most of our vodka, we decided to check out the play areas with them. Once there, they decided it was time to part ways, and I sat down next to an attractive single woman who seemed interested in us. We talked for a bit, and she seemed more and more interested in exploring some fun with the two of us.

Just then, the couple we'd been chatting with reappeared, and she took an immediate interest in the woman I was talking to. So much so that she decided she'd sit down between us to get the woman's attention. What she didn't seem to ascertain was that there was just empty space between me and the single woman. Expecting a barstool to be there, she attempted to sit between us and landed on her ass on the floor. When the woman reached out to help her off the floor, her ring broke in two and went flying across the hallway. She looked rather perturbed, but then she said it hadn't been expensive, and not to worry about it. Tyler and I sat there, stunned by the turn of events. We thought surely she'd made enough of an ass of herself that the single woman would return to conversing with us.

The woman did just that, and began to ask us some questions about our sexual predilections. She asked if I go down on women, and I said yes, I do. At that point, the other woman jumped back towards us and practically screamed, "I go down on women! I'll go down on you! I'll do it right now!" Looking a bit taken aback, the single woman shrugged and replied, "Well, how can I refuse that?" The two disappeared into a play room, and that was the last we saw of them.

Tyler and I sat there, once again in stunned silence over the strange courses our nights tend to take. We wandered around the club a bit more, then we decided it was most certainly time to head home before any other strangeness took place. While it often seems we look around a club and see everyone but us happily hooking up, apparently we're not the only ones who swing and miss, sometimes repeatedly.

We seem to strike out every time we go to the swing club and try to meet couples. We find a cute couple and introduce ourselves, and we will talk for an hour or so, and everything seems to be going fine, then another couple with more "game" swoops in, charms them, and lures them away. It's like school dances on crack and steroids at these places! I think we're destined to be the wallflowers.

~Gina, Denver, CO

A while back, I drove over three hours from Tampa to Jacksonville to meet a girl who said she was dying to meet me...when I got there, she said "no thanks" in a round-

about way...and I headed home. Still don't know what

happened.

~Ben, Tampa, FL

I like the proposed title for your book, because my wife

and I feel like that's what happens to us all the time – we

swing and we miss! We go on dates with other couples two

or three times a month, and it leads to sex maybe one time

out of nine or ten. This isn't the image of swinging you get

from documentaries and talk shows! I don't know if it's

just us, but I don't think it is. I've heard similar things

from other people in the lifestyle. I think our friends who

know we swing imagine we're hooking up with random

strangers every time we leave the house, and swinging

naked from chandeliers at wild parties. In reality, for us, at

least, it's not so different from dating.

We like to know and actually like the people we engage in sexual activities with, so I suppose that makes it a bit more complex than just hopping in bed with whoever happens to be at a club. That's not our style. We'll meet a couple that seems incredible, then my wife notices brown spots from smoking on their teeth, or they say something mildly racist, or any number of things, and it's over. We do this for fun, it's not a necessity, and we need to feel good about people if we're going to get naked with them. I'm sure the reverse happens as well, although we never know what it was that turned people off. There have been a few times when we met a couple, thought it went great, and we never hear from them again. With all the idiosyncrasies people have, it's kind of amazing four people are ever able to all find each other attractive and otherwise acceptable enough to sleep with!

~Jackson, Long Island, NY

We went on an early anniversary trip to Chicago a few years back, and we happened to make contact with a very sexy couple in the area before we flew out. We emailed back and forth, and they seemed extremely nice, laid back, and similar to us in many ways. We made plans to have dinner our first night in town. They were nice enough to offer to meet at a restaurant just around the corner from our hotel, and we thought that boded well for some after-dinner fun. We had dinner, and it was great. The conversation flowed, and we all got along really well. They suggested a bar up the road, and we went there afterward.

It seemed we'd all be on our way to the hotel after a drink or two. As we left the bar, the couple wished us good night, said it had been a long day, and suggested meeting for dinner again the next night. We certainly understand long days, and while we were disappointed, we took it in stride and looked forward to the following night. We'd

actually made tentative plans with another couple, which
we canceled, as we felt this was definitely going to work
out. We met for dinner the next night, and once again, as
soon as dinner was over, the yawns began, and they said
they were tired from working all day and needed to turn in.

They mentioned a big party the following night, and it
was finally the weekend, so a late night was possible. It
was going to be our last night in town. Again, we agreed.
We made our way via bus and subway to the party location,
and they showed up a little bit later. Conversation was
once again great, drinks were flowing, and things seemed
to be on the right track. We were attracted to them both,
and the feeling seemed to be mutual. Then, out of the blue,
around 1 AM, the male half approached us, hugged us, and
told us he was heading home, and that his girlfriend was
staying to dance. We were stunned.

We had no idea what had happened to derail the night.
We told him goodnight, hung around with her another hour

or so, but we felt very uncomfortable because we just didn't

know what we'd done wrong, or what had happened.

Finally, we told her good night and headed back to the

hotel. We were baffled and a bit irritated, to be honest,

because we spent three evenings with this couple and felt

they sort of led us on. Not that we MUST have sex with a

couple we like, but our time there was brief, and we spent

quite a bit of it with them.

I got up the next day to pack and get ready to head to

the airport, and to my surprise there was an email from the

male half of the couple awaiting me on my phone. I must

admit, I expected some sort of apology for his flakiness and

for pretty much ruining the fun for us all. Quite to the

contrary, his email was a long, rambling "what the fuck"

sort of tirade, berating us for sending mixed signals and for

wasting their time and wasting a good opportunity.

While I'd been disappointed the night before, at that

point I was ready to throw my phone across the room in

anger. I had no idea what in the world was going through his mind when he typed that email, OR, for that matter, the previous three nights when we were ready for fun and he seemed ready for a nap. After calming down, I sent a rather harsh, but civil, reply. We emailed back and forth for an hour or two, and by the time we arrived at the airport it appeared to be some huge misunderstanding.

They had been waiting for us to make a dramatic first move, and that's not our style, and I suppose we were waiting for more signals from them, signals which we never detected. By the end of the correspondence, we all felt a bit better towards each other, and I think we all felt quite foolish for not just being more up front from the beginning. We all wasted a pretty good opportunity. And I still regret that.

~Shane, Santa Fe, NM

We just had the strangest "date" with a couple. It started out when a couple who lives about an hour and a half away emailed us and wanted to get together. They said they would be happy to come to our city and meet us, so we made plans to get together for drinks. From their photos, she was quite beautiful, and as my wife said, she'd have to see the guy in person to know for sure how she felt. But based on how pretty his wife was, we were willing to meet them and see what happened. After looking a bit more closely at their profile, we realized they currently live in two different states and spend one weekend a month together.

We thought that was odd, but we figured we'd maybe get together with them for fun next time she was visiting if all went well over drinks and conversation. We even figured we'd make the trip to them, rather than having them drive back to us. Anyway, we met them and they were delightful. She, in particular, was bubbly, outgoing, and very down to earth for such a gorgeous woman. We were impressed. He kind of let her do the talking, but he seemed charming and sweet as well, and we were impressed with them both.

During our conversation at the bar, though, they began to talk about their grueling work and life situation, and it came out that she only comes to see him every other month, and he goes to visit her every other month. He also mentioned he would be relocating in a few months to be with her full time. We both gave each other a puzzled look, but at that point what could we do but just proceed with hanging out with them and try to figure it out later.

My wife and his wife both went to the restroom, so during that time I decided to try to determine why they'd made this date with us if our schedules would likely never align in order for the four of us to get together again for playtime. In talking privately to him, it became clear he'd

been looking at our profile for some time, and he was
interested in getting together with us on his own.
Apparently, when she's in town, she "helps" him meet
couples so he has some diversions while she is away.

Well, we do meet with single guys from time to time,
but I felt absolutely duped by this situation. My wife never
would have gone for this guy for a threesome; she was only
willing to give it a chance because we were both
immediately attracted to his wife. It felt like a big-time bait
and switch. Of course when our wives returned, I couldn't
say anything, but I was honestly ready to end this date.

We talked for a bit more, then we decided to head out.
My wife suggested going to another bar up the street, and I
cringed. She didn't know what I knew, and she was still
thinking there was a chance for the four of us to hook up.
When we got to that bar, it was a bit too crowded for
everyone's tastes, so I took the opportunity to suggest that
it was time to part ways for the evening.

Once back in the car, I asked my wife what she thought

of the guy. She seemed somewhat nonplussed by him but

said she was opening to meeting them again. Then she

mentioned their weird schedule and wondered aloud how in

the world we'd be able to get together with them anyway.

She asked, "Why in the world did they drive all the way

here to meet us when there's probably no way they'll both

be down here again before he moves away?" Well, I told

her about my conversation with him, and she just about

flipped out in the car.

As I said, we're more than happy to meet respectful

single guys for fun; if he'd presented himself as such, we

may have met him on his own and had a great time. What

we don't tolerate is dishonesty or shady behavior – and

that's what we feel happened. He felt he could lure us in

with his super-hot wife, and then we'd find him charming

and want to get together. Unfortunately, it was quite the

opposite. He blew it big time. Big missed opportunity on his part.

We spent literally three hours hanging out with a couple at a swing party several months ago. We had seen their profile online, and they said they'd seen ours, but we hadn't talked until that night. The conversation and chemistry were great, and we were all flirting, being touchy feely, and enjoying the vibe. The husband suggested we find an unoccupied room, and we all agreed and went in search of a room. It turned out a private room with a locking door happened to be open, so we all went in, shut the door, and sat on the bed. Sometimes there's a little bit of awkwardness before the clothes start coming off, but this was ridiculous. They went from talkative, flirty, and touchy to shy and reserved, with a deer in the headlights expression. I scooted closer to the woman, hoping to start off the action, but she immediately jumped up, grabbed her purse, opened the door, and was gone. Her husband shrugged, apologized, and said they'd see us later. When we composed ourselves and exited the room, we walked around the club, and they appeared to be gone. We're not sure what happened. Major case of cold feet, we guess. But it was a downer. We only go out every few months, and this was not how we anticipated that particular night ending!

~Becky and John, CA

In swinging, just as in regular dating, things simply don't always work out. Attractive couples often have things go awry, or they strike out despite their best efforts. After five or so years of observing swingers in "their natural habitat", the swing club, I've determined that the couples who hook up with people every single weekend are a distinct minority. At the risk of sounding judgmental, it seems those are the same couples who aren't terribly interested in *each other*, so perhaps they work a little harder than the rest of us to make sure they find someone else to have sex with when they go out. And, also from my own observations, they seem willing to lower their standards to do so. The rest of us are more than happy to simply go home with our own significant others should nothing interesting take place at a club or party. I'm thankful to be in that group!

Epilogue

Well, there you have it. Stories from swingers across America who were kind enough to share their own experiences with us. Perhaps these stories were not quite what you expected; perhaps they're just what you thought they'd be. The general public has varying perceptions of what swinging means, and what swingers look and act like. We're all different, and from my own observations, swingers fall into many of the same cliques and social groups that the rest of society does; they merely socialize with somewhat different intentions. Unlike the portrayal offered by cable documentaries, though, swinging is not a "home run" proposition, with horny couples participating in orgies every chance they get. The pitfalls of dating, rejection, issues, drama, and inexplicable weirdness befall swingers more often than they'd like to admit. And once again, the truth I've discovered within the swinging world is much, much stranger than any fiction could ever hope to be.

Turn the page for an excerpt from Audra Morgan's swinging memoir, available exclusively on Amazon.

An Excerpt from Swinging by a Thread: The Misadventures of an Accidental Swinger

Prologue

I've read quite a few "memoirs" over the years which were quite obviously exaggerated to the point of becoming complete fiction, with only the smallest grains of truth scattered throughout. I'd like to point out, straight away, that this is not such a story. Much of the past five years of my life has fallen into the "truth is stranger than fiction" category, and a dear friend downright insisted I record my strange, but true, stories so that my life could serve as comic relief for someone other than her. At her behest, I've done so, and other than changing names to protect the far-from-innocent, all of the details in the pages before you are my own true, unembellished life experiences. In fact, they're so accurate that I'm bound to get an angry email or two from people who recognize the stories a bit too well! Still, I felt compelled to tell these stories, and to keep it real. For some of you, it will serve simply as the means to a good laugh. For others, it may hit close to home, reminding you of some of your own funny experiences. For others still, it may even spur you on to create some adventures of your own. And if you do that, I hope to read about them one day – I could use a laugh that isn't at my own expense!

Chapter One

How It Began, or Always Blame the Bartender

This is the story of five years of crazy adventures in swinging, and of some of the things I've learned through our more outrageous encounters. You don't know me from Jack, so I'm not going to bore you with a twenty page background on my life. Still, I think context is pretty fundamental, so let me begin with a little bit about *us*, and about how we ended up on this path.

Tyler and I spent the first ten years of our relationship being homebodies. He was never much for going out; he preferred a quiet night at home, watching movies or playing games. I, on the other hand, had to adjust to the quiet life. I'd spent my years in college and grad school partying almost nightly, and my new, quieter life was a big change, to say the least. I grew used to it, though, and then once we had kids, it became a no brainer that nightlife from there on out would involve falling asleep watching Saturday Night Live together. Yes, the all-too-typical routine of being married with kids. With that routine, though, came a serious emotional and sexual rut in our relationship. For a while, we both assumed this was the natural progression of marriage; it seemed everyone we knew was going through the same thing, so we didn't discuss it, much less attempt to fix it. It just *was*. At some point, we thankfully agreed that our relationship was worth more than that, that we were *better* than that, and we began making a conscious effort to change things for the better.

For our ninth anniversary, Tyler surprised me with a night out which consisted of an amazing hotel room, dinner, and a fun night at my favorite bar from my college days. It felt so good to get out again, to be around people drinking and laughing and having fun. I felt like I'd come home, and Tyler could see how happy I was. From that point on, we made going out at least once a month a priority. We settled into a wonderful new routine of meeting our friends, mostly the parents of our kids' friends, for cocktails and dancing and general absurdity. Monthly nights out turned into twice-a-month gatherings, and those nights were soon supplemented with drunken game nights and movie nights. We were truly having more fun than we'd ever had before, and our marriage was all the stronger for it. Then, one night, a bartender at that very same bar told us a story that, quite honestly, changed our lives forever.

Gene, our favorite bartender, smiled broadly as we entered the bar one Saturday night. He made us our drinks before we even reached our barstools; we were pretty predictable. As he placed our drinks down on the bar, he leaned forward and began to tell us about his adventures the previous night. "Guys, I have to tell you about this club I

131

went to with a friend last night. It was insane. Naked people everywhere. Having sex! I've never seen anything like it. You guys should check it out, you would die!" Before he could tell us more, he was called to the other side of the bar, and that was the last we spoke to him that night.

Now, I've never even been to a strip club in my life, it just holds no interest for me; I'm a naturally curious person, though, and it intrigued me that this place existed in my city. This club with regular people who got naked and had sex in front of each other. Did these places really exist outside porn and bad Tom Cruise movies? What kind of people would go to such a place? Had Gene been exaggerating, as I suspected he sometimes did when telling stories? The next morning, despite my hangover, I was up early, searching online for answers to my questions.

"Did you know we had a swingers club here?" I asked Tyler incredulously. He'd heard a coworker talk about it once, but he didn't really get any details. I still couldn't quite fathom it. Unfortunately, what we could find online just didn't quench our thirst for details about this club that had been operating for nearly ten years mere minutes from our house. While I'd never had any desire to set foot in a strip club, I suddenly felt a need to have a glimpse into this secret world where things happened that I had to admit I couldn't even really imagine. Regular people, exposing their bodies and their sex lives to others, not for money, but for the sheer enjoyment of it. I felt like the most sheltered, naive person in the world, and I felt the overwhelming desire to unburden myself of that naiveté.

Now, let me make one thing clear, in case you weren't paying attention: Tyler and I were not, had never been, and had never considered being, swingers. We'd been monogamous, with no exceptions, for our entire marriage, and we had no intentions of changing that. That being said, we both felt drawn to this mysterious club, simply so we could see what went on there, and so we could be "in the know" about this secret place that apparently did not even have a sign on the door or a listing in the phone book. We quickly realized that if we were going to learn anything about this place before actually stepping foot in the door, we'd have to make contact with people online and get information first-hand.

We emailed a few people who had posted in online forums about the club; we made it clear that we were just going as visitors, to check the place out, and that we wanted to learn more about it before we actually went. A very nice couple replied to our email, told us all about the club, and assured us that people are more than welcome to just go, have a few drinks, check out what was happening, and leave without having to worry about being accosted in any way. In fact, they pointed out, we were more likely to be hit on inappropriately at any random bar than at a swing club. Who knew! This couple was from out of town, but they'd been to the club many times before; they offered to meet us a few blocks away at a neighborhood bar, walk us to the club (since it was somewhat difficult to find), and show us around. We appreciated their kindness and generosity, and we made plans for that weekend. We agreed we were going simply to drink, people watch, and learn a little about this completely different way of life.

For the rest of this book, please look for **Swinging by a Thread: The Misadventures of an Accidental Swinger**, *only on Amazon!*

Printed in Great Britain
by Amazon

28951681R00079